How to seduce a girl in seconds

Content

Guide on how to pick up a girl in a few seconds

Flirting with a girl effectively is anyone's dream, especially since it can shorten any time to get to know her thoroughly, even convince her to go on a date and put into practice some detail of seduction, if you want to get to this level you need to discover the actions that yield great results on women.

The ways of flirting can generate an idea for you to gain confidence, this is a basic point to take care of, because it is what allows seduction to flow effectively, until you conquer the girl for real, start by discovering the techniques that will facilitate any situation before a girl.

The best flirting techniques and what doesn't work with girls

The seduction techniques with the best results can be applied to avoid any fear, or in an uncomfortable situation, the important thing is that you can stand out and that is the intention of implementing methods for flirting, where psychology is the source of knowledge to find behaviors that cause the expected effects.

But when you follow tips or methods for flirting, you must take into account at all times the type of situation in which you find yourself, that way you can be totally useful strategies, so the essential thing to develop is a reading of what is happening, without leaving aside the fact that compliments never fail.

About women it is important to express to recognize her beauty, from what she wears, to her way of being, that will always be a classic way to be remembered in a positive way, so you should not omit this kind of details, but the dynamics vary for each type of woman, so flirting goes hand in hand with those aspects and the recognition of the following techniques:

1.   Attention to the smile

Most men are captivated by the smile of women, but it is a gesture that can be taken into account as a striking detail to highlight, although it can be overshadowed by certain negative signs such as shyness, so a man should keep the look towards the smile.

2.   Listen carefully

An action that cannot be missing when flirting, is the ability to listen which is highly valued in interpersonal relationships, this strengthens all types of social ties reaching a much more intimate point, especially in view of the data showing that women talk more than men.

The data described above has been scientifically proven, since women have a higher protein load that has a direct impact on language, for this reason their need to communicate is a biological aspect that you can take advantage of.

As you are attentive and can listen to her needs, so will you receive attraction from girls, that kind of characteristic cannot be overlooked, the more value you implement, the better the girl will feel, being in the company of someone who really listens to her.

3.   The attractive side of intelligence

There is no doubt that an intelligent man is striking for a woman, but without reaching an extreme where the excess of this quality can intimidate the girl or even be a sign of ego, this is part of the personality and how you make a connection with other people, which requires a little more humility.

4.   Humor

A desirable aspect in any seduction is humor, as women are interested in being made to laugh, because that means she can spend pleasant moments with him until she wants to repeat an outing, but this also includes being able to get him to find the humor behind the jokes.

These points are essential to produce a pleasant feeling, but at the same time to get a next date, because they are details that a woman wants to repeat to feel good, but there are other aspects a little more superficial or external that you can also take seriously to get the attention of girls:

- **Odors**

The effect of scents, is a highlighting power for any date, which works to achieve a really striking impression, every woman emits an assessment regarding the scents, beyond any physical quality, this detail remains on their considerations, and is a much easier resource to manipulate just by choosing the right perfume.

A woman perceives a man in a better way by what he is able to emit his perfume, there is no doubt about the attractive side of the smell, it is a signal or direct stimulus that has an impact on the brain region, at that point visual information is also processed, so it has an effect just as relevant as a good look.

The processing of scents ends up being a point on which you can take advantage, you can even choose some that have pheromones that work to create an attractive impact on the opposite sex, so it is a measure on which to invest very safely.

- **Concentration on the eyes-mouth triangle**

An important trick in the middle of the tension of flirting, is to dedicate a deep look on that triangle eyes-mouth, this is vital to be held in the middle of the conversation, as it is a way to awaken some sexual feeling, some women can also interpret it as a sign of desire for the other person.

- **Repeat your name to personalize the conversation**

The unique treatment towards a woman, can be highlighted by maintaining a direct treatment on her name, this is a psychological aspect, since each person develops a narcissistic side by nature, which indicates that he/she wants to feel valued and a way to show it is through recognition in every conversation.

Every time you emit the pronunciation of her name, you will gain a liking over the girl, so start repeating her name when you are addressing her, it is a powerful way of seduction because it links an important social bond.

• Group tactics

It is usual that when flirting you want to spend more time in intimacy with the girl, especially to gain more interest, but in the case of the first contacts, it is best to appeal for group plans, since there are social virtues that stand out more in group stays than alone.

• Interpretation of non-verbal language

Discovering the techniques of reading nonverbal language is very useful, since you can measure the receptivity of your actions as you interpret postures, these types of manifestations, work as an evaluation of interest, the same happens with what you emit, since crossing your arms for example denotes a level of insecurity.

A common mistake is also to look at the type of position that has the head, when it is an irrelevant fact, because what does work as a reference of interest is the posture of the torso, as well as the position in which the legs are, another gesture or known signal is touching the hair, as it signals different emotions of a woman.

These signals beyond allowing you to interpret what is happening, can also be a message that is issued consciously or unconsciously to capture your attention, so these details can not be overlooked to make a change of conversation or generate a rapprochement.

These points mentioned above can not be considered infallible, but at least you can start from the basis of scientific research, as they focus on studying the mind to measure the above signs of corporeality, these aspects allow you to try to take control when flirting, but there may be exceptions on these points.

You can not forget that seduction is an art itself, it is developed as a personal strategy, from each recommendation you can bring a sign of your own personality, so you can succeed in this action to conquer a real girl.

Shyness as a flirting strategy

In the midst of the tricks to flirt, you can come across a personal trait of being shy, but this condition is very profitable when it is focused to your benefit, in cases of need or interest to conquer a girl, is when the wit comes to the fore, so there is a seductive side over shyness.

Nowadays through technology, it is usual to meet girls through a screen, being a trend that is gaining ground over any outing to the bar, but instead of detracting from communication, it is considered a more effective way to avoid having to go through the usual tremors.

This implies that, for shy people, technological imposition is a wide scenario of opportunities, so these tools to meet people can be used in the right way to achieve results, since a much more controlled social context is ideal for shy people.

Through an application, the whole dynamic of getting to know each other becomes more controlled, since even awkward questions can be put aside or be dispelled with an emoji, all through simple buttons, leaving aside that main problem why they did not dare to flirt.

The impediment to meet new people, has been left in the past since they can flirt freely in chats or draw attention through social networks, being an environment where you must bring out your wit to enliven a conversation, so this creates an opportunity, but for this means of seduction to work:

1. **It's not a question of how but where you can recruit.**

The main advantage of using an application, is that forming a relationship acquires a simpler approach, but this must be combined with other ways, i.e. you can meet her remotely, until a time when there is a real date, it is an evolutionary perspective on seduction.

Social interaction is a resource that should not be lost, since even social networks allow a type of exposure that can be striking for a woman, so you can gradually move on to enjoy different emotions on a face-to-face level, that way everything is facilitated by having a previous knowledge of the girl.

2.   Going out in a group

To challenge any level of shyness is positive to rely on a collective outing, especially without a previous appointment, you can bet on meeting and stand out from the circle of friends, that way you can be on a date, under a much more social atmosphere, it is the advantage of fitting in with friends of my friends.

This method to meet and flirt with girls is classic, because you can be in front of your next partner without meditating or taking it into account, so they are details to which you should pay attention, that closeness of a social circle is a much more pleasant context to put aside shyness.

You don't even need to plan, you can simply take advantage of the office, and even sports activities, the medium doesn't matter, it should only be crowded and allow you to meet more people without forcing it since they are part of the same social circle and you won't have to strain or feel uncomfortable.

3.   Knowing what to say and prioritizing listening skills

The secret to diminish that shyness trait, is by practicing what you can say, or at least managing dialogues in your mind so that you have more confidence, no matter how the approach with a girl takes place or where, the vital thing is that you keep a natural essence, but without sounding out of place.

A first contact always implies additional actions, i.e. it is a stage for your skills to come into action, beyond shyness, you can get an interesting moment when you put in place topics or open answers, thus the situation starts to be in your favor.

On a first date or other outing, it is best to follow the standards of these meetings, so that the interesting capabilities are those that guide every moment, instead the limitations you can try to reduce them for that day, ie shyness can be overcome as long as there is confidence with the girl and you see advances of yourself.

4.   Expresses compliments that excuse your limitations

In the face of some embarrassing behavior because of your shyness, you can dissipate that moment in front of the girl, by exposing a compliment like "excuse me, it's just that you make me nervous", that eliminates all the tension of what you have done before, besides it is a sign that you care, changing the course completely of that scene to a seductive environment.

For any shy man, it can be complicated to appeal for the lip to flirt with a girl, but with phrases of this type that are simple and take all the pressure off you, you can be much more relaxed to conquer the girl you want, this has a great margin of influence on the conquest, since it is about using your weaknesses as strengths.

5.   The ability to listen is increased

Faced with the difficulty of expression, there is nothing like devoting all that energy to listen attentively, getting to discover the positive traits of that girl you want to flirt with, beyond having an episode of embarrassment, you can say nothing and look at her to start getting all your attention.

Letting your non-verbal language take control of the situation is easier, because no matter if you are not talking, you can opt for a more sincere seduction, it is effective to pay attention to these actions, because it is an easier terrain to dominate, to use in your favor that knowledge about the girl.

The most brilliant ways to flirt according to expert studies

The opportunity to flirt, is not accessible to many, first of all, by the high degree of shyness, as well as the lack of confidence in yourself, all this in general line is to go adopting a habit or appropriate behavior before the girls, allowing you to face any situation with your personality afloat.

Through self-help books many men can find answers, especially to overcome the difficulties of seducing a woman with all the confidence possible, this means that for the most part it is a step that requires techniques and a personal vision, because seduction is unique to each man.

That is, what works for one man, may not work for others, so some may succeed and others fail, so these are recommendations that should not be seen as a magic key to 100%, but can be viewed as methods to better address a situation according to your interpretation.

At the moment of seducing, the type of girl you want to seduce, the environment in which it develops, as well as the mood you have at the time of establishing a bond with her, all these external factors play a role to consider, so each tip should be assessed according to the way in which you adapt.

- **Work on your mood level**

This has to do with the formation of a pleasant personality, this can be confused with seeking in every instance to be funny, when in fact that image also ends up tiring a girl, so what you should aim for is the emission of more witty comments, being a rapprochement and consolidation of the social bond.

A simple way to get to socialize with a girl is through jokes, but it requires a criterion to choose the right time as well as the type of comment, so you can reach a better effect, the essential thing is not to reach the extreme of tiring the girl.

In some boring circumstances, you can break that atmosphere with a joke, since it is part of the ability to surprise the girl, without leaving aside that it is a good action to capture the attention in the middle of the seduction, shortening some awkward silence that may arise.

But before making a joke, you can keep it natural by saying it slowly without any nervous gestures, and the type of postures you are presenting, because they should stimulate the level of enthusiasm, much less you should choose to change the subject to talk purely about you.

- **Don't limit yourself when it comes to praise**

The use of compliments is a double-edged action, it also requires greater care, because the best method to use it is through an intention to break the ice, it can also be a way to generate closeness, thereby presenting feelings of empathy to chain a natural conversation.

Making qualities acquire a level of recognition is a great way for the psychic aspects to make an impression, i.e. your intentions can be brought out through the right compliments, leaving it up to the woman to accept whether she reciprocates those compliments in view of what she feels.

You must keep in mind that there are limits to use compliments in the right way, where you can measure the moment through non-verbal language, the essential thing is that there is no excess that is annoying or that is used to attract attention, in that process for nothing in the world you should expose your own virtues.

Although before a compliment or praise, you can also expose yourself to some negative reaction, so it is a step or advice that is unpredictable, especially because every woman will interpret that praise differently, so there is no guarantee on this resource, but if you receive before any negative, it is vital that you do not present some insistence.

- **Presents a friendly and attentive attitude**

There is no doubt that an attentive attitude to lend support is highly valued, when there is a sign of this willingness you will generate a liking on the girl, this feeds a positive atmosphere in the midst of seduction to the point of being seen as reliable, so in every occasion you have, you must express that willingness to want to help her.

Instead of asking, you can bet on having a much more resolute attitude, that really impresses because there is not such a forced environment, this implies that you should not rush, but keep a composure not to fall into excesses, that way you will not lose a positive result.

When wanting to do a good deed, it is not necessary to fall into a momentum with so much ego, much less is it effective to look like a cold person, so what should be appealed to is an attitude that is classified as a gentleman, although this depends on the generation and the level of culture of the environment.

The secret to making seduction work

Getting a girl to melt for you is feasible by following the right advice, without the need to choose the best outfit, much less postulate yourself as the sexiest before the girls, the balance is just right, not to fall into an excess of intellectual personality, much less with the ego at 100% where money is imposed as a priority.

In order to completely conquer a woman, it is crucial that you do not abandon subtlety, along with other fundamental rules so that you can give the best possible presentation, that way you can fall in love with the girl you want, but with the respect of indicating that you are not looking for something serious beforehand, if that is the case.

Building a relationship based on sincerity is the right thing to do, so you need to follow the following actions that will help you get the best results:

1.   Seeks contact or approach with hands

A woman wants to have or feel closeness through contact, this is possible through the hands, as they can imagine a lot about you, just by seeing your hands, so you can start adjusting your accessories or try to show your hands as much as possible, either writing something or playing an instrument.

As you use your hands in front of the girl, she will be able to realize how they are, these can be used as a symbol of attraction, in this way you will attract your girl, causing her not to stop looking at your hands until she finds herself surrendered at your feet.

2.   Every woman loves to have her hair kissed

This is a very simple step with great meaning, although for men this has a paternal definition, but women love it because that kiss in the hair or on the forehead causes them to feel a great protection, so when there is confidence you can exhaust this way to get to meet a dearer feeling beyond the physical.

3.   Behave like a gentleman

Every woman loves that a man can behave like a full gentleman, so the details on how to open the door, this should be fulfilled so that your company can be more pleasant for you, that way you can issue a striking presentation as a natural offer, being a help for him to want to be with you.

4.   Value its natural facet

A woman really appreciates that she can be loved with her face freshly lifted or without makeup, this becomes a compliment for any woman, so you can awaken that kind of appreciation, it is a sensitive sign that can be exploited to have a seductive closeness on the woman.

Above any sexual tension, it is essential that the stay with you can be associated with a much more attentive relationship, that way it is much easier to take the moment to a more intimate moment, so the level of closeness by sharing a more natural image, can be exploited to the fullest.

## 5.	Always look her in the eye

The eye contact is an ideal way to approach any woman, you can try it to convey ideas and feelings, but without abusing it because you can fall into an extreme of intimidating the girl, the intention is that you do not look like a stalker, so that it does not present a nervous reaction, but rather seek a seductive effect.

## 6.	Take care of the level of communication

Every woman loves to talk, so as a man you must maintain a very fluid environment to generate a high level of trust, so that feelings and concerns can come out or be expressed, being emotional aspects which opens the way to a lasting connection.

When you make a woman feel fully heard, as well as a reciprocal response, it gives way to a friendly atmosphere, she will want to go out with you again, this is important and is tested on the first few dates, you need to work on this aspect so that you are desirable in the eyes of a woman.

How to overcome embarrassment and pick up a girl

Some men find it difficult to flirt, either for reasons of shyness or other, this problem can be set aside, so that when you get to that point of looking for a girl, you can achieve greater success, managing to reduce the barriers that exist to meet a woman that attracts you to form a relationship.

The ease or means to establish conversations, is a skill that is achieved progressively, because beyond flirting, it is important that you do not lose the focus of meeting people, because the essential thing is to enjoy and have a good time, to the point that you can relate with a greater degree of security, to lose the fear you can conquer.

- **Bet on your personality**

It is essential that your personality as a man does not change depending on the date with a girl that you attend, because when there are some advances it will not be interpreted as authentic, because later it will expose your true way of being and it may not be pleasant for the girl.

A golden rule is to avoid lying about yourself, much less with what you do or your age, this only gives off a bad image of you, this way you will not get very far in meeting the girl, since at some point the truth will come out, so in the future everything can turn into chaos.

- **Put the enjoyment of the moment first**

Flirting plans need to go hand in hand with fun, since after each invitation the ideal is to prioritize having a good time, that at the same time decreases any intention of seeing you as a simple hunter, also a woman values the intention you show to meet her, rather than just a sexual or direct objective.

Abandon such an invasive posture, leave aside that empty treatment so that naturalness is the main thing, especially because you're going out with a girl you like and that should be noted in the attitude of having a good time, the same happens if you go out alone, it is better to focus on exploring the place and what you can do, no matter how much you can flirt.

It's okay if there is no breakthrough on that occasion, the best thing to do is to remember the experience and always emit a high liking of the girl's company, that way you lessen the obligations to make it a fun scenario, which in turn makes you look more charming, as you prioritize the time and living with her.

• **Think about your physical appearance**

In every outing it is essential that you present yourself with an appearance suitable for the context, as well as a much more conscious personal reference, it is not so much about investing in clothes, but in hygiene, neatness is a seal that women value widely, instead any unkempt sign only causes rejection.

Men's grooming encompasses hair, beard, and any other details you can adjust before going out, you should think about using some cream that can boost the kind of look you convey, the essential thing is to achieve a much more radiant style, as those personal traits are left or esteemed much more than some muscles.

A man beyond any rude personality, must also have a care for what it emits, there is no excuse for neglect, since it is only a basic step as is hygiene, and the second is some complement as a perfume to reaffirm that essence, without excesses of any kind, neither in care nor in perfume.

- **Select relaxed plans and avoid discom-
forts**

When you are organizing a date or a plan, where you have some expectation of flirting, it is vital that you take care of the mood of the moment, this includes even the type of food you choose, because some women may find it uncomfortable to be with a man who is eating garlic or who is drunk.

Composure is a key point, unless there is a much more advanced level of trust, because there are details that even with chewing gum or care you will not be able to avoid, even your friends may feel annoyed by these gestures, you should not abuse the trust that exists, since some aspects are related to tolerance.

- **Play with the seductive power of glances**

In the midst of forming relationships, one way to create a close atmosphere is through looks, it is simple and can lead you to get a nervous laugh, or some kind of reciprocation, this action is so crucial that it is believed that when it fails, there is not much to do to get the girl's interest.

The crossing of glances reaches a much more tempting and attractive approach, because it is able to awaken any level of spark, the next thing to do is to mention some phrase that can second a physical step, the eye contact helps the girl can think that she is receiving your full attention.

The only measure to consider is that they are not aggressive or intense looks, in addition to managing the type of context, since when you are among friends that kind of attitude can be classified as misplaced, the main thing to measure is that you have the opportunity to reciprocate that look with a smile.

- **Creates pleasant topics of conversation**

The incorporation of interesting topics is ideal, because you can get their opinion, as you also get to know each other completely, it is a much more mutual line that releases the pressure of flirting so that it becomes a pleasant moment of conversation, for this you can look for a common ground or a passion.

A negative action that you should not do for any reason, is to bring up topics that generate conflicts or are extremist, such notions only complicates that you can meet her, and she may even dislike any position you have on a topic that she is passionate about, so it is advisable to be receptive and bring up open topics.

On the other hand, getting involved with familiar topics without any kind of confidence is also not a useful ground, so a more generic category is placed on hobbies, type of music or movies of your preference, the essential thing is that on the topics do not present know-it-all attitude, and stay willing to learn from that contact.

Infallible actions that every man should know

To flirt once and for all, leaving behind the obstacles, you need to master certain techniques that are useful for men, since the action of conquering is not a simple step, and the first thing you must fight with is the lack of confidence and shyness, this is what makes any seduction strategy meaningless.

When flirting becomes very complex, there is no doubt that you can bet on a much more effective help, it is an appropriate guarantee for you to take that definitive step, which is framed through the following tricks:

1. Use your sense of humor to the fullest

Humor is a fundamental quality before women, for this reason it is so insistent with the fact of causing grace to a woman, especially when looking for an escape from the routine, for this reason a negative man has no chance at the time of flirting, in fact, is exposed to receive rejections constantly.

But when it comes to humor, it is not about using it to the extreme, moderation is useful so that it does not become a trait that is so exhausting, so jokes in excess are totally out of place, the bet should be persistent on naturalness, that way inopportune gestures are diminished.

2.   Maintain a cordial attitude

Politeness is a sign and a way of being that you should try not to lose, because a woman does not seek to be in a serious way with a rude man, much less when they are just flirting, which forces kindness to be a persistent requirement, being an attention that makes any woman feel good.

A woman's appreciation for this type of courtship is unique, so you can concentrate on the basics, such as avoiding interrupting her, then accompanying her, because this translates into attentive care, but keeping the limit not to overdo it.

The chivalrous side of a man should not be overpowering, otherwise it loses all kind of shine, and even comes to be received as a meaningless action, the essential thing is that you are not overwhelming with the girl, in addition to avoid at all costs to present a macho behavior, because they are attitudes that will not lead you anywhere.

- **Postulates a sensitive treatment**

The sensitivity of a man is a huge point of attractiveness, so by showing that you have that kind of vision you will approach women easily, you will only need the treatment to be sweet, that way you can be more attentive to emotional level, but as long as you feel comfortable to have this position.

Sensitivity can easily merge with security and strength, as they are elements that shape your personality, which goes hand in hand with that masculine side, you can't hesitate to strike a balance of this so that it comes through in your behavior until you are the center of women's attention.

- **Without manipulation and with naturalness in every action.**

When flirting, no situation should be forced as this only increases the possibility that you push the girl away from your side, so any false attitude when detected only pushes you to receive rejections, so a response that does not fail is the naturalness, so that in every contact there is sincerity and a relaxed treatment.

No lie, no matter how much argument you have, will be well received for flirting, a base built on falsehoods, will only end up triggering a chaotic outcome for both, this indicates that overacting is an enemy not to incorporate on your relationships, so that you reach a much more enjoyable conquest.

- **Respect their space**

Contact with a woman should not start with an intense encounter, this is a common mistake especially at the beginning or when a relationship is not yet mature, it is serious because it reduces the freedoms of both, respect for the space of the other is an issue not to overlook.

In order not to generate some kind of emotional fatigue on the girl, you should avoid interfering with her routine, but bet on being part of her environment, without invading too much privacy, that level of relationship is pleasant so that at some point she misses you and has the initiative to ask to see you.

- **Don't forget originality**

Monotony when flirting is a common enemy, so the original seal that you possess as a man, helps you get a privileged place and confidence on the girl's life, it is also very limiting that in full seduction emit a compliment that has been heard and published millions of times.

The plans of conquest should not overlook the diversity of options, it is vital that you can propose to do something different, especially what involves having a good time, to keep the atmosphere alive you can think of including surprises, this is key to gain more dynamism to the girl.

The tastes of both are the ones that should drive the direction of the relationship, also in each phase of seduction you should take everything calmly, it is better that everything is flowing instead of issuing pressure, the processes of conquest require a breather so that the moments come to be remembered until they want to have you as a partner.

How to be successful during dating

Understanding the most important details in dating is a step that can open many doors to flirt without so many setbacks, until you get a greater number of positive responses that are hopeful for your future love, for this you should consider these measures:

- **Diversify your strategies or places to pick up**

It is essential that you do not take everything for granted when flirting, that is, there is no perfect way, but you can consider other measures, so the horizons should be open to more options that allow you to flirt with girls naturally, a mentality that only pushes you to look for meeting girls at a party, limits you from other possibilities.

You never know for sure where you can find love, so a more open vision facilitates the process, you must play all your cards to flirt with a woman you really like, especially when there are so many women waiting or looking for a conqueror, so you must have your eyes more open and willing.

Wherever you go there is a great situation to meet girls or friends, this can be at work, on the street, in the cafeteria or any kind of public environment, all are an opportunity itself, but you should consider these key points:

Interacting with a girl in a supermarket can be a complicated activity, because most of them attend a context without an additional purpose, but they are dedicated to fulfill their goal, so you must be tactful with what you try to flirt in these environments.

-Popularly indicated as a favorite a night environment, since a large number of girls come with a clear purpose to flirt, or at least to have a good time, so you can blend in better among people, without it being a requirement itself to have to flirt with a girl.

The most recommended way to start conversations or go out to meet a girl, is through markets and outdoor environments, this causes it to be a more receptive environment, to the point of establishing much more reliable conversations, what matters is to enjoy and at the same time take care of details such as a sign of interest.

-Some men use as a rule of thumb to present themselves in a crowded area, wearing a ring that provides a more interesting style, this is much more focused on mature men, but otherwise when you observe a woman with a ring is better not to insist if there is no initiative from her, as you expose yourself to a clear rejection.

- **Study in depth about emotional relationships.**

For each country can be established as a standard, some traditions about the type of relationship that is developed, but you can also customize this research, where you get to clarify some paradigms that you have about relationships, gaining emotional intelligence, which is very useful to know how to act when flirting.

One of the most classic questions is to find out what a woman likes or is attracted to in a man, so you can get an idea of how women's minds work, and by incorporating it with your personality, you can exert a striking social power, there is always a lot to know about emotional issues.

Generate a better social impression is possible, all thanks to the power that generates information, a much more conscious treatment towards what women want, is a high degree of attractiveness, thanks to the fact that you can develop a gentlemanly style and full of humor that is successful, but above all that they get to emphasize their strengths.

An essential way to gain confidence when flirting is to inquire, social power through information is recognizable, which helps you gain the ability to establish conversations to have a reliable behavior, leaving aside fear, which is very powerful to be attractive to a woman.

- ## **Bring out the best version of you**

At no stage of a flirt can you seek to win a girl with falsehoods, as their personality is very perceptive and at the same time sensitive, so they can detect a deception and hardly overlook it, it is a lack of respect and commitment to be pretending something you are not.

At the same time, a negative version of yourself, does not leave much to be desired about a woman, because they are not looking for a man to fix their life, so in the long run you should work on putting aside worries and fears, that way you can be a better match for any woman.

The perspective when seducing a woman should be fixed, but without the need to talk too much or exaggerate about any seduction strategy, it is best to keep the kindness of a good treatment so that there is a real interest.

- ## **Positively enhance your body language**

There is no doubt that an element or aspect such as body language, is an element that counts and you can start wor-king from standing with your back straight and maintaining full eye contact at all times, all this should be located in the same package, the essential thing is that everything that involves communication is improved.

Body language is a transmission of many details to keep in mind, being a signal that can become mutual, for this reason it is a way of communication to value, while you can learn about this demonstration, you can get better results on a date, so put into practice the following rules:

Increases the level and stability of eye contact, an excess of eye contact may be more passable than a lack of eye contact.

Look at her and smile, in the middle of the eye contact you must accompany it with a smile that can make the environment more enjoyable, no need to look away or much less, the essential thing is that the smile does its thing.

Do not stare, what should be practiced is that the eyes do not become fixed on your body, since at the beginning the attention should be located on the conversation.

Keep at all times with an open posture, for this you should reach a relaxed arms pose to hold the legs without crossing, in every circumstance the shoulders should be back, with the leveling of the head at a stable level, in this way you can emit a reliable presentation completely and receptive.

-Work on your communication, because a gesture like stammering only takes you away from the attractive pose, so the goal is to speak with total clarity, otherwise it can be interpreted as a dubious personality.

-Stand with an inclination close to the girl, as you possess interest to talk to the girl, you should keep attentive and close, in case you are sitting you can seek to stay closer to her, as the faces aligned.

- **Consider the confusion of body language**

In the middle of a date, just as poses are important, in the same way you can highlight a part of you by touching it with your hands, on the other hand, also adds the interpretation of the gestures that a girl emits, because in the case of touching her lips when talking to you, it can be taken as an insinuation.

A woman's interest can be gauged by this kind of observation, it is an important incentive, although sometimes it can be simply itchy, so any clue should be taken with calm.

- **Every action counts**

At the thought of determining whether a girl is interested in you or not, the right thing to do is to take the situation into your own hands, because that is better than waiting for three years or living with eternal doubt, that is, by not acting you get to feel or experience a large margin of adverse consequences.

The slowness to win a woman's heart can be a negative aspect to deal with, especially because in most cases it doesn't work, especially because women wait for a man's boldness, so when you have the opportunity to say what you feel, you can't hesitate.

The demonstration of interest in a girl, is a continuous action to capture it on each date, to reach that point you must overcome the fear of rejection, you just need to find the right opportunity.

-Modern women do not like to wait too long, but must be met with an active invitation, so a decision to act must be presented, regardless of whether it is attractive or not, it is vital to keep the courage so that you can ask her out, and even take the next step to an approach.

When you are attracted to a girl, it is essential that you wait for the right moment to present another invitation, as it is better to postulate your intentions progressively, the perfect timing helps to preserve the charm.

The most effective methods to flirt with a girl

When you want to flirt and get the results you expect with a girl, you must consider every detail especially when you do not externalize that desire, the basics is to issue an invitation to simply talk, it is essential that you maintain persistence and you can use the following steps:

1.   Organize a list

Before flirting, you can create a list of your concerns regarding a girl, this can be lack of topics, lack of plans or the discomfort of an environment, by developing this list you are going to be able to focus on overcoming adversities, an initial base allows you to take that leap or push to act.

2.   Take care of the fluency of a conversation

An entry in the middle of flirting, it is essential to create it under the conversation topics that are presented, where you should avoid receiving a cold response, but when it happens what you should do is to desist from this idea, to post a last attempt to flirt, because it may happen that the topic you are bringing up does not fit the context or intentions.

On the other hand, when you receive from the girl, some warm or compatible response, you should let the conversation flow naturally, that is the way to have a much more passionate development.

-There is no doubt that a big challenge is to hold a conversation with someone you barely know, but as long as the topic of conversation gets easier, she will be able to participate in an open way, where you can include inconsequential opinions, such as highlighting the type of music in the environment, without detracting from the honesty of the topic and going into more detail.

Try not to turn the conversation into an interview, so some questions such as what you do for a living, where you live or where you studied do not have space, because they may be irrelevant to the emotional issue, and much less appropriate if they come from a quick succession that transforms it into harassment, it is better to go spontaneous.

3. Take advantage of humor

A universal language with which to fit in with others is through humor, the feeling it conveys is very positive, but there are types of jokes for each person, as not all work the same, so you can go measuring the situation until there is a situation of pleasant response, using humor as a subtle approach.

-No matter what kind of conception you possess about your sense of humor, you can try to let it out in the middle of a conversation, you can gauge whether to stop or continue by the girl's laughter, plus when there is interest involved she is going to be sympathetic to sustain the mood and make you feel better.

4. Compliments should follow a subtle level

Every compliment you give must be expressed naturally, that is what sustains a fluid conversation, and in case any disjunctive arises, that kind of comfort to debate is generated by the trust built, where you can insert some compliment without stopping the conversation, it is a minimal flirtation with punctual phrases.

The response you should expect from a compliment, is that the girl agrees or accepts it, so you should not judge or position yourself to evaluate if it is self-centered, nor if she is ashamed of it, she may even want to return the compliment, the essential thing is that you communicate how much fun you find her presence.

5. **Demonstrates your willingness or dispo-sition**

A girl does not like to date a person who does not possess self-confidence, much less who does not answer your questions honestly, so love or attraction for sensitive guys who are focused on their interests and possess a permanent smile for doing what they like, without being ashamed of it, may prevail.

-Do not avoid making some criticism, you can subtly add your point of view of something like; Don't you think it is exaggerated or extremist, you can vary the phrase, but you can leave the question open to know what she thinks, you can also make jokes that are kind because a guy can be attracted, but not dazzled, you can help her to improve.

6. **Ask for their number and stay in touch**

Once that crucial moment of ending any encounter arrives, it is time to ask for her number, home address, social network or anything that keeps you in touch, which at the same time reaffirms your desire to see her one more time, this you can add with a statement of how much fun you had.

The plans to see her again, are exposed when you emit that desire to share with her once again, in case she does not provide you with any communication data, you should not stop being polite, but when you generate a positive response, you should take into account waiting for a reasonable time to schedule a next appointment, so you do not look so desperate or disinterested.

7. Get in the right mindset for a good first date

A good date is one, where you do not spend too much time together in silence, because interaction is set in motion, but this does not mean that you should choose places where there is no opportunity for a conversation, such as it happens with cinemas, concerts and so on, the best in any circumstance is a space to talk and get to know each other.

At the same time, it is not appropriate to choose an expensive place just to impress, as you may be conveying the wrong image of you, to decide better, you can create a list of ideas and alternatives that meet a great time for both of you, especially since women prefer the man to organize the dates.

If you have any additional ideas while on the date, such as going skating or renting a car, going to the movies and so on, that can be a good suggestion, but it depends on your mood and how the situation is going, but the least risky is to follow the classic as a lunch or continue with a coffee, the essential thing is that there are options to continue spending time together without getting bored.

-Offer to pay without insisting too much, in the traditional means of gentlemanly gestures, it is usual to hold the invitation until the bill is covered, so choose the place should be adjusted to your possibilities, women love this conventional image and others will want to pay split bills, it is best to issue the comment and see what she prefers.

Don't invade her space too much, on a first date space is a sense of respect to preserve, because you are not going to marry her at that moment, so from the beginning when the date is scheduled, don't call insistently, especially when you are going to meet that same day, it is better to have something to talk about in a personal way.

When you receive a change of plans, you must leave open the benefit of the doubt, because in case of a full rejection, he would have called minutes before and without the option to leave another day, so this communication of rescheduling should not be taken badly if not be patient and measure their interest.

How to flirt with a friend

When you want to flirt with a girl, there are many inconveniences involved, but when it comes to a known woman like your friend, everything changes completely, since there are more factors involved so that a real connection can arise, where you must keep in mind the following aspects:

- **Reasons the risks**

There is no doubt that this seduction situation is one of the most delicate, but you can keep in mind that normally she would not stop being your friend just because you have asked her out, even if she does not want to go out with you, the problem arises when she expresses a refusal and you do not accept it, but you seek to ask her out again.

On the other hand, when you issue a normal invitation as friends, the girl may think that you continue with a higher interest than that of a friendship, so when you possess any desire to date your friend, you should consider that you expose yourself to possible rejection, and even disappointment that you are no longer friends, there are many scenarios.

- ## **Wait for some time alone**

So that you don't have the fear or possibility of some embarrassment in front of mutual friends, you can look for an occasion that is more intimate for both of you, that way regardless of the facts, you are going to feel much more comfortable, there is no need to go through a moment full of heartache if you are patient.

- ## **Issue a simple invitation to go out**

Instead of issuing an awkward declaration of love, you can leave everything on friendship terms by just asking her out, regardless of whether you love your friend, if you express those kinds of feelings, you're not going to change anything because you're not conveying a reason to go out with you.

It is best if your feelings can be kept discreet, so that you can visualize the plan to go out as just another usual offer, without any kind of commitment, until you boost your chances.

Be careful about showing your interest in inviting her on a romantic date, the best thing is that a simple date to spend time together prevails, although when you are very obvious it will not be enough to hide what you feel, as this may even create some confusion.

- **Retains control of the situation**

Regardless of how the offer of a date has been, you must keep as a general rule to continue with a mature and polite treatment, this is a responsibility so that you do not damage the deal you have with your friend, although it is part of the risks of this type of taste, and when she says yes, you still need to have composure, first of all.

The first date is not yet done, so calm is an indispensable way, before any refusal you must avoid feeling the need to retaliate, but rather apologize, avoid crying over the rejection, as this may be a way to force something that she does not feel.

How to flirt with a coworker

In the work environment an inevitable social interaction develops, this can lead you to want to flirt with a girl who is part of your work team, but at the same time it is a complex choice because it can alter the future of the work environment, to take that definitive step, you can take into account the following measures:

1.   Analyzes the risks

There is no doubt that, in a work environment, some possibility of flirting with a girl is real, but at the same time it is a risk, since in the face of a positive or negative action you are going to work close to her, which can be uncomfortable, so every detail counts in the midst of this type of seduction.

The level of comfort you wish to maintain at work is a factor to be considered, as there may be results to be taken into account, so you can take care of developing measures to diminish the negative impact.

2.   Take into account the saying "don't defecate where you eat".

This saying has been applied throughout time, for each country has some variation, but its meaning is clear, as it implies that the closer you are to people who are not related to the love bond, it will be much more pleasant to go out on a date, otherwise being with her can be a total drama and remain immersed in stress.

In work matters, this only indicates that you can do better to flirt with a girl who does not have to do with that environment, or at least who is not so close to you frequently, being another aspect that you can avoid to avoid falling into some boredom or problem of coexistence.

If you don't work in a big company, you can make it a rule to pick up girls from another department, that way there won't be so many circumstances to deal with, this lowers the level of discomfort because she will be in a different environment than you, so there isn't as much stress about the outcome.

3.   Emits a respectful attitude

Respect is a fundamental element to sustain any type of relationship, and in dating this takes on greater meaning, so when dealing with a girl related to the work environment respect is key, therefore each proposition should be estimated from her point of view, that is to say thinking about how she will take such a proposition or comment.

On the other hand, you know the girl by the simple fact that she attends with a willingness to work, not with an intention to look for a guy, so you have to be careful, the same thing happens if it is a very stressful environment, she will not want to go out with someone who reminds her of that place, it can even be interpreted as continuing to work.

It is crucial that you don't cause the girl to be afraid to go to work because of running into you, so before you ask her out you can gauge what kind of future the relationship would have, or if she is a girl who has the same vision about a relationship or a passing flirt.

-In the middle of the conquest of the girl do not fail to be polite and concise, especially when there is some refusal to go out with you, there is no reason to fall into some kind of insistence, but to continue with a friendly treatment, since insisting very rarely is appreciated, as they may not really be interested, and everything becomes annoying.

4.   Act with discretion

Before any invitation to go out, you should also consider that some colleagues do not like to be in an environment of romance, much less when the purpose is that there is a work development, even for superiors this is seen as a decrease in productivity, or goes against the accepted behaviors.

Because in the middle of a work scenario, distractions may arise because of that conquest, as well as work stress because of the breakup, so before asking out a girl at work, you should try as much as possible to make your intentions not so noticeable.

One key is to maintain the same dynamic or way of working when conquering or dating the girl, that way the environments will not be mixed, this prevents the bosses from having any disagreement with the fate of that conquest, also appointments should be kept with a regularity that does not alter the work environment.

Don't forget that, in the work environment, the most important thing is the work, everything else is of secondary importance, no matter what happens with both of you in the relationship, this is an attitude to keep.

Tricks to flirt with a girl when you are traveling

An opportunity to open yourself to adventure is being on a trip, so if you meet a girl, you can consider flirting with her using the appropriate techniques and tips to succeed in this attempt to change your emotional life.

- ## **Analyzes the type of dynamics of a travel romance**

A trip can have the motive of a family enjoyment, as well as a full fun, in the middle of that dynamic you can find yourself in a coffee shop or a local with a girl with whom you can date in the middle of that adventure, it is also a way to not spend those moments alone on your own.

When traveling abroad or within the country, you can discover each environment with better company, where you can consider the option of flirting, since it does not represent a problem itself, because while you are traveling you can maintain a much more pleasant treatment, to live every moment that offers the transfer, but without taking it as one more or something passing.

- ## **Shows a much more direct attitude**

You can't face flirting with a girl, when you are willing to lie, much less you should hide some kind of information, this will only create a false bond and will not do much good for both, especially because more intrigue generates flirting with a person who is just passing through on a trip or as a contact that arose spontaneously.

The best thing about this kind of relationship is that you don't have to submit to a premature commitment, but that you both recognize that you are in an adventurous situation and the possibilities are more open.

A trip itself is a topic of conversation, so it is a simple scenario to establish a relationship, there are no problems of running out of ideas or something similar, so the traditional efforts are left aside, with mentioning some detail or place you are visiting, it serves to approach the girl.

- ## When flirting with a girl you must be quick

In the middle of a trip, there is no room for any shy attitude, much less to act demurely, if you want a date, a night out or to meet her, you must take the necessary steps for it without postponing it, since you run the risk of not seeing her anymore, besides she will not know the kind of interest you possess for her if you do not show it to her.

Instead of going slow and just asking for his number, you can suggest a date on a tour of the trip, that way you can also bring up a topic of conversation where he suggests places to visit and vice versa, to think of another next approach, the key is to maintain a posture of adventure and at the same time flirting.

- ## Do not hesitate to remain faithful

When you have a girlfriend or someone waiting for you when you return from the trip, for no reason should you seek to have something with a girl on the trip, as it is a cowardly attitude and at the same time it is unfair to the girl on the trip, because she can realize and chaos is created in the middle of the trip, it is a heavy issue for your conscience.

It is the same as if when you come back you find out that your girl went for a weekend trip with another man, or on the contrary, she kept missing your company, so do not put at risk any relationship, or play with the feelings of both, because everything can end in an emotional disaster.

In any case where you want to end your relationship because you have meditated during the trip, the ideal is that first you can put aside that link to be able to open up to another, it is useless to act behind the backs of both girls, being single you have more opportunities to act independently.

Tips for flirting with a girl in any circumstance

Beyond the scenario or the situation in which you find yourself, flirting becomes an art itself, since every performance counts and the impressions you can generate are in full expectation, to leave aside the pressure that exists in this process, you can apply the following tips:

1. Practice every tip

The practice of the mentioned techniques is what will turn you into a master of seduction, or at least increase your chances of success with women, since you will have an important contribution of security, which allows you to get rid of fear, until you get to have a woman relationship with women.

To have a better perspective when flirting, it is worth to know and inquire about the formation of relationships, being a way to get along more feasible, this helps you get used to have that kind of contact without nervousness, which facilitates communication completely leaving aside the intimidating aspect.

2. Issues a balanced treatment

You should always treat a woman as your equal, because when you take it upon yourself to give her a superior role you will only emit an attitude of an inferior man, therefore you should not put her above you, this does not mean that you should treat her badly, but that you can build esteem in a subtle way, instead of doing it by flattering her.

3.   **When you want to get an appointment**

When you want a date to manifest itself, you can choose to explore different ways, either by a website or a dating app, even social networks work as an ideal way to do so, managing to find out what interests him and gain an advantage with him, so nowadays there are plenty of ways to start a conversation or flirt with a girl.

4.   **Act loose**

The impression counts, but also the way you act, so before a woman you should not present yourself with a fear or a totally robotic way of being, you can be nervous but control is everything, the good management of a date will help you to project who you really are and also the girl can feel confidence in you.

5.   **Expect a reciprocal gesture**

Interpretation plays a key role, so when you issue any phrase or action, keep an eye on how to react to take a second step, this helps to not become a much more uncomfortable situation, it is essential to keep these measures when flirting, it is not necessary to assume that you must please him.

No girl is interested in hints, much less confusion, so at all times you must appeal to clarity and a good understanding, in some scenario on which you impress her, you must let time do its thing so that she emits a natural reaction to you.

6.   In the face of the desire to flirt with a girl with many suitors.

Some girl with a suitor, you can get her attention over others by staying positive, and above all gentlemanly, there is no reason to compete or show any anger, if not enjoy her company so that she can develop an attraction for you, this is a way to consider not to suffer too much in this process.

What to avoid when flirting with a girl

The following recommendations are some measures that will reduce the risk when flirting with a girl, you can carry out these prohibitions:

- Do not stare at the girl, the best thing you can do is to pay attention to the location of her eyes, instead of observing another part of her body that may confuse the deal between the two, everything is possible except stares, as it can be uncomfortable at a certain point.

- Do not emit an impression of insecurity or authoritarian, since that kind of personality only decreases your chances of conquest, girls do not want to meet a man who behaves like an animal, on the contrary, they want to have a good time and enjoy, the intention is that you emit good reasons.

- Don't show off as a pick-up artist, appearing before a girl with that intention only generates an impression that you do the same with others, besides following planned attitudes limits your daring personality, this causes that the most appropriate thing is to follow a voluntary path without so many impositions.

Techniques that girls love

Spending too much time online, is generating two kinds of behaviors on men, firstly, there are the men who are too sensitive that they do not move a finger, waiting for the love of their life to knock on their door, or on the other hand there are those who flirt by publishing a much more liberal facet of themselves.

That is, this last way of being, expresses that men are dedicated to publish much more threatening content to look attractive, these two images do not group 100% of men, but it becomes a common denominator in the opinion of women, so the methods of seduction should stick to what a woman craves.

When you generate more frank approaches, you can escalate to a more erotic state without having to force a relationship so much, handling more romantic ideas is what will allow you to open up to what a woman longs to find in a man, especially to expose that not everyone is the same or has these visions.

To find a woman who really feels something for you, you must focus on the expectations that exist around a relationship, because it is not about behaving without any conscience, much less forcing her to have something with you, but the opposite, you need to know her to really conquer her.

The first step you should take is to investigate each scenario, that way you can adapt your romantic mode to the environment and to the girls themselves, because every personality must be tolerant to form a real bond, understanding that the interaction when flirting is an action of two.

1.   **Social networks and dating applications**

It is usual for most men to keep stalking or following every post of a girl they are interested in, the same goes for using Tinder, as you may come across some eye-catching profiles that you won't want to unsee, it is a modern game to get to date through digital ways.

The strange thing is that you get to get a strange attitude, where you dedicate yourself to see the profile of the girls for more than 15 minutes as an obsession, as this has nothing healthy, plus you should not fall into an empty side of only look at the superficial, that behavior is usual to be in loneliness or despair.

You should not call yourself an enthusiast, and then put it in your profile as looking to generate some attraction, because those words will not be a substitution or description of your personality, besides a girl is not interested in that, so it is better and more explicit to publish a full body type photo, it all depends on your qualities.

In the case of Tinder chats, you should avoid bringing up conversations about plans to celebrate the weekend, or any other generic topic, when the best step you can take is to ask her out directly, that way you limit all the effort to simple steps, instead of banalities, it is best to create more open plans.

• What they want to talk about in person

Normally men get used to talk the same thing they talk to one, copy it and paste it with another, but when you talk in person everything changes because it uncovers your true personality, especially since some girls love to be talked to, but it adds the factor of considering the environment, since they do not want to flirt just anywhere.

It is important that in the middle of a conversation physical approaches are also developed, because every woman at some point in the seduction just want to be the man who can take the step, but without losing the charisma as well as the essence of the moment, because without igniting the moment you should not make any choice.

Another key point is that, if you have conversations about your private parts, do not show them in photos, far from it, physical contact is what is worth more, so the most advisable is that you can have an approach taking advantage of the circumstances, otherwise you can get more rejections online.

• Women love home parties

In any part of the world, a single woman, loves to take a break from society, so a party is an ideal way to get intimate with a girl, but under a home environment can gain a much more tense atmosphere, as there are more options to bring seduction to another more physical plane.

A house party usually lowers its level at 4AM, the rest is about to happen according to the opportunities you have for you to have a more sensual approach, it is the dangerous side of this kind of environment because tiredness can lead you to emit a bad image to the girl, so you can save some phrase for that moment.

What you should keep in mind is optimism, because bachelors are the ones who have the most fun and possibilities at a party, so you can relax until you wait for the final outcome to approach the girl.

- **What they expect most in bars and nightclubs**

Beyond some home partying, mature people prefer to go to bars and nightclubs, as they can go with a circle of friends and avoid any interrupting, it is an environment to experiment better to flirt in public, especially to have the freedom to take advantage of alcohol.

No matter what type of personality you have, there are bars for everything, for smokers or to go dancing to Latin music, this also helps you get a girl that suits what you like to do, this is useful for men who have a good rhythm of conversation, as well as a captivating body rhythm to ask her to dance.

On the other hand, talking at the bar is feasible to get to know in depth that girl you are interested in, or you can help someone who has more than 5 minutes ordering at the bar without being served, that kind of detail leaves an important mark so that chemistry can flow more easily, the rest is to smile and go with the rhythm of the environment.

Don't hesitate to introduce yourself at the slightest opportunity, because a woman wants to get herself with that kind of initiative, chivalry is still valued above feminism, even if you can just approach to talk about how rude they are at the bar, it's a more subtle form of support without going over her head.

In the midst of this environment, there may arise the doubt about how to determine if the girl likes you, the usual is to measure the reaction of her friends, you can also visualize if she has been signaling you all night, to this is added the fact of assessing whether she has a friendly face to seek to touch her arm to approach.

- **Linking in a private area**

To find love, you must be willing to try in any environment, so you should know that an ideal place is to start a conversation in the smoking area for example or in a more secluded area, because they are areas that are kept in the dark most of the time and can help you level up.

In the case of not being a smoker, for example, do not hesitate to pretend, because it is an open door to flirt with girls, before some lack of opportunity, you can approach those who are holding the purse of other friends, as they are types of women who love to be taken out of that boredom.

Offer her a drink or a cigarette, the ideal is that the good vibe that exists in that club or area, this brings life to any kind of conversation, also translates into a good deal so that the girl can be amazed with the way you are attentive, you can even look for a lighter for her to continue smoking.

There is nothing more uncomfortable than a moment in silence, that's why these environments make everything easier, either with a cigarette or a drink, but this should not boost your ego for any reason, but you need to keep a feature of attention on the girl, as this fascinates her completely.

- **Become Prince Charming in front of his girlfriends**

Once you have isolated a girl, when you are flirting in a group, you should not underestimate the opinion and effect of the environment, because the group is also an influence itself for the girl, so you should stand out in front of them, especially if her best friend is present, because they act overprotective and may judge you.

For this reason, so that no one interferes in your plans, you need to focus on treating her friends in a special way, as well as the girl in front of them, so the main thing is to make clear your interest in only one so that there is no disagreement between them, knowing that you want to flirt with her friend, they will focus attention on both of you.

Once you are talking, you should not make a mistake in mentioning some jokes, do not even try to convince another one when you have failed with the first one, or lastly, do not make an insinuation about a threesome, because you are together, you barely know each other and this makes it a huge risk.

A more advisable measure is to be nice to her friends, it is not about flirting, if not that they like you, to the point that they feel jealous of this interest, so you must maintain an active conversation with them, you can help you deciphering which is the leader to make yourself noticed by her.

Having her friends on your side is an ideal advantage for flirting, instead of just throwing you to the criticism that may arise, so do not hesitate to be affectionate or attentive, but in a sense in which she can notice it, that way you will be estimated in a positive way, standing out in that way opens the doors of a seduction influence by her friends.

The ideal phrases to start a chat when flirting

Thinking like a woman, is a posture that men should adopt, to get to flirt more easily, you also understand how key it is not to lose an attractive image on the girls, as well as you must maintain care about what you express, this is what differentiates you from the rest of the men who have met and rejected.

Stealing a woman's heart, being a lout, is definitely not what they are looking for, this idea is very little enjoyed, plus it falsely feeds self-esteem, you should always care what girls think of you, especially since it is a sure way to generate a level of provocation over the girl.

Instigating a woman's curiosity is a feasible action, but without getting to the point of being intriguing, that is the personality you should postulate when you are in full chat with a girl, otherwise you can emit an image that you are out of reach of any girl, being just the opposite you want to get to seduce a woman.

Most women know what the games or techniques are all about, that is to say that if there is any answer it is because they themselves want to advance, so you cannot take them for naive at any time, much less can you judge the experience they have, this reinforces the idea that you should not issue any false information.

1.   How to add the idea of a girl's performance

The turning point when flirting with a girl, is how to bring up the subject of sex in full seduction, this depends on measuring the balance of the situation to make it a more delicate event than expected, to reach that point, avoid incorporating a phrase so direct that it breaks the atmosphere.

Instead of expressing something dirty, you should let everything flow so that you don't get a rejection reaction, because there is a big difference between tickling and you telling her something dirty enough to want to run away from you, on the other hand, when you think about moving the date to your apartment you should express it clearly.

There is no need to experience fear in the middle of a date, you are already in front of the girl and there is not much left to think, because all potential flirting requires will, to measure the times you can question yourself if it is time to kiss her, but before acting remember to propose something and thus go acting subtly.

Any movement must follow a natural destiny, leave for later the nervousness, do not rush the situation because you are not buying something in a store, it is a matter of reading, as well as to keep in mind the limits that you have, so you can have the patience that is needed in those moments.

2.   Don't ruin the moment in your apartment

Once in your apartment, it is time to act, there is no reason to delay the physical advance, much less when you have been talking for a long time, if she is in your apartment is because she is attracted to you, what comes into play is the aspect of the setting, where you should avoid doing something that cuts the passion.

This means that in front of the girl is not the time to change the sheets, unless you distract her, on the other hand, do not fall into the temptation to give her a tour of the house, since she did not come to see your property, but to have a moment with you, it is an environment where you must be direct and continue.

Similarly, if your room is too messy to break the passion, it is better to stay in the living room, because otherwise you can undo everything you had achieved that night, if you have musical instruments is not the time to demonstrate your ability, it can serve later to make it more enjoyable.

In the midst of seduction there is no need to rush the dynamics, this means that it is not recommended that you express that you are not looking for something serious, that way you can flirt and raise the intimacy of your partner without any problem, it is an achievement of moments without hesitation or persist when the time comes.

Techniques for flirting with strangers

You need to keep in mind that, when flirting with a girl, an aphrodisiac measure is not presented, but techniques are implemented that yield results because seducing a girl is not a simple task, many men would like to study this topic in depth, as the level of usefulness is high to incorporate a philosophy of attracting the girls you want.

It all starts with a guy meeting a girl and from that moment on you can develop a whole series of actions that can ease your way:

- **Behave as if you were on vacation**

When you are on vacation you dedicate yourself to explore everything with curiosity, as you also insist on meeting people, this same attitude is associated with flirting, the best thing is that this opens the doors to fun and surprising events, in the same way you should dare, just as you would while traveling offering a drink.

This way every time you go out, you can psych yourself up with a similar view, you live in a wonderful city to explore, by looking at everything through a different lens you can expand the opportunities for you to notice the women around you, you may be overlooking some interest.

• Get rid of routine

In the middle of each week it is vital that you break the rhythm, you have the control to achieve it, you just have to think of something you have not done, that way you can have the will to go to places you are not used to visit, especially if they are susceptible to meet people and even allow you to flirt.

• Frequently attends restaurants

When you go to lunch, you can think about attending an open place, since this is part of your routine and instead of being boring, it can be transformed into an adventure itself, because lunch is an opportunity to meet women.

• Go out alone anywhere

It is not a great idea to go out in a group to flirt, it is better to approach a girl or a group of friends on your own, that way you can also get to know her better, because a woman may feel intimidated in front of a group of men or think you have a girlfriend if you go out accompanied by a woman.

- **Smile most of the time and stay friendly.**

As you walk around on your way to work, don't hesitate to smile at everyone, it's a gift that no woman will be able to resist, she may be watching and feel attracted.

- **Consider going to the gym**

A tempting side of a man, is to highlight that sporty and attractive side, and there is no doubt that a gym is the ideal environment to postulate yourself as a great candidate, you can meet a lot of girls, as well as friends and you will take advantage of getting in shape.

- **Go to crowded places and queue up in lines**

To talk to girls in a casual way, there is nothing like taking advantage of a queue, this applies to the cinema, as well as the supermarket, this helps to dispel fear, using any topic of the place as an excuse to approach.

- **Go to bookstores**

To find a cultured woman there is no better way than betting on a bookstore, where you must appeal to a purely literary seduction, this helps you when you go down the road and see a girl with books, you can consult what she is reading and thus expose your knowledge in these areas to seduce.

Discover how to flirt on WhatsApp

To fall in love with a woman through WhatsApp you can use seductive messages, nowadays there are many ways to exploit when it comes to seduction, it is also a starting point that is used to take physical contact to another level, as long as you do not use it to hide, it will be a tool that you can take advantage of.

1.   Don't be tempted to send too many messages

A key rule in the midst of seduction, is to maintain a minimum flow of conversation to ask her out, also going around in an invitation does not generate many benefits, it is useless to hide your intentions, but in the chat you must be direct and concise, that way you avoid being in the friend zone.

There is no need to bet on long conversations, being in contact is very simple, now the complex is to move to another level, no need to fall into more problems, just seek to increase the desire of the other person, and leave aside the tension, the course to follow is to demonstrate a passion as if you were seeing her every day.

2.   Think twice about what will be the first message you are going to send

A key step in the middle of the conquest, is the emission of the first message, and at the same time is an action that is not much thought, so you should take time to take that step, at the same time you must consider that the messages are limiting to expose how you are, and if other men write you will be one more in the pile.

You need to be clear that in a chat you should not try to sell yourself, but rather keep a masculine expression within the first message, where you should not make mistakes, that distinguishes you from others, to increase your chances you need to send natural answers.

A clear example is to tell her that you are interested in getting to know her better, take it slow to respond, and test her interest in a different way, or in the face of some hidden meaning it is better to ask for explanations than to just assume, preserve honesty and generate an open-air conversation to stoke the passion.

What is not recommended is to think too much about what to answer, or blame yourself for not getting an answer, or that you have done wrong to provoke a bad reaction, nor should you write too much, do not exceed three lines, you should not even talk about everything, or send photos to show off.

3.   Don't always be available

This advice may go against your interests, but it is essential that you reach a level above which you make yourself desired, that way your masculine energy gains more value, to flirt with a girl on WhatsApp you should focus on your life and then see if she fits with the kind of life you lead, and not the other way around.

This also applies in the case that he writes you, it is not recommended that you respond so fast, you must also have an attitude of being busy, it is complicated and you may feel afraid of losing it, but it is something you must learn over time, just visualize it from his place, if he has interest in you you can provoke him to call you.

An action of this type is considered as a strategy to seduce, besides forming a relationship without losing your emotional independence, the mobile is an appropriate means to awaken that desire, this helps to overcome the attachment for the result, the fear that everything concludes, omission of a net sexual desire and waiting for a change that may not come.

It's a matter of becoming aware of yourself, it's an opportunity for both of you to really get to know each other, without giving too much importance to the girl without having something concrete, by putting this into practice you can focus on yourself.

4.   Don't waste time thinking too much

When you are writing to a girl, you should not put your life on pause, because this only causes you to overthink and collapse in the face of a bad outcome, this only helps your anxieties increase when she is not responding, that loop is harmful to your confidence, nor should you think that she is only writing to you, because it is a delusion far from reality.

Around you there are many activities to follow closely, commitment within your life is a common trait, because every woman wants to find a determined man, it is a very harmful mental process that falls short with the appropriate measures, on the other hand, it is not necessary to have in mind some physical change to please him.

One way to distract yourself is to go out with your friends, there is no better medicine than a friendship to distract you from the evolution of the flirt with the girl, this increases your masculinity, the support of activities and external people is key for you to get where you want.

5.   Measure your interest when flirting with her

The interest of a girl can be sincere or false, so it is a resource to measure, especially in WhatsApp where there is no real interaction, so that you distinguish what she is looking for, you can leave conversations in suspense, but be careful not to run the risk of losing her, and before an intention to only go out for casual sex, they should make everything clear.

To test or measure a woman you can apply as a technique the fact of not responding for two days, or try to tell her openly that you like her, in case of any sexual interest do not hesitate to be clear, and in case of any net deal as her friend, do not hesitate to confront her.

www.ingramcontent.com/pod-product-compliance
Lightning Source LLC
Chambersburg PA
CBHW061515250726
48657CB00005B/1884